The Art of Breast Play

Mastering the Techniques, Psychology, and Pleasure of Breast Play for Enhanced Intimacy, Connection, and Fulfillment in Your Erotic Journey

Cheryl Bach

The Art of Breast Play

Publisher: IntimateInk Press

Email: intimateinkpress@gmail.com

This book is a work of nonfiction intended for informational purposes only. The content of this book is based on the author's research, knowledge, and experience, and it is provided with the understanding that the author and publisher are not engaged in rendering legal, medical, or professional advice. The information in this book is not a substitute for professional guidance or assistance. Readers should consult with relevant professionals for advice and assistance regarding their specific situations. The author and publisher disclaim any liability for any loss or risk, personal or otherwise, which is incurred as a consequence, directly or indirectly, of the use and application of any of the contents of this book.

Cover design by IntimateInk Press

Interior layout and design by IntimateInk Press

Printed in USA

Fonts: Google fonts

Image: Freepik.com. This cover has been designed using assets from Freepik.com

For permission to use copyrighted material from this book, please contact the copyright holder listed above.

First Edition: 2024

Distributed by Amazon.com, Inc.

Cheryl Bach

Table of Contents

Cheryl Bach

Chapter I.

Introduction

A. Overview of the Book

The Art of Breast Play: Mastering the Techniques, Psychology, and Pleasure of Breast Play for Enhanced Intimacy, Connection, and Fulfillment in Your Erotic Journey is a comprehensive guidebook to help you master the various techniques of breast play. This book explores the psychology of breast play, the importance of communication and consent in sexual relationships, and the benefits of incorporating it into your erotic journey. It's a must-read for couples who want to deepen their intimacy and connection during sex.

B. Importance of Breast Play in Sexual Relationships

Breast play has been around for centuries; it's found in almost every culture, and for good reason. Breasts are an erogenous zone for many people, both male and female, and they have tremendous potential for sexual pleasure. Breast play can be done at any stage of sexual activity, from foreplay to intercourse, and can enhance intimacy and connection between partners. For some, it's an integral part of their sexual arousal. Whether you're new to breast play or a seasoned pro, this book is designed to help you master the art and explore its many facets, from teasing and tantalizing to full-on pleasure.

In summary, "The Art of Breast Play" is an in-depth guidebook, covering all aspects of breast play from the psychological benefits to foreplay, sex positions and incorporation of toys and accessories. It provides insights into enhancing pleasure, connections and emotional intimacy with your partner during various fondling techniques. With this guide, readers can discover and

Cheryl Bach

master techniques that will help them enhance and expand their sexual journey.

C. What Is Covered in the Book

In this book, we explore the topic of breast play from a psychological and emotional perspective. We discuss why breast play is important to people of all genders, what types of breast play individuals may engage in, and the implications it has on an individual's emotional and sexual well-being. The book emphasizes understanding personal preferences and boundaries, communicating openly with partners, and fostering a respectful and safe environment.

Additionally, we address societal stigmas surrounding breasts and their sexualization, promoting body positivity and self-discovery. This book provides a comprehensive guide to exploring the potential benefits of breast play while ensuring an inclusive, respectful, and safe experience for all individuals involved.

The Art of Breast Play

Chapter II.

Understanding the Psychology of Breast Play

Breast play may seem like a simple sexual activity, but it has several psychological implications for individuals and can be an essential part of their sexual experiences, regardless of their gender and sexual orientation. This chapter aims to explore why breast play is an important part of sexual exploration and how different people enjoy it.

A. Why Breast Play Is Important to People of All Genders

Breasts are an erogenous zone for many individuals and have been found to activate the same areas of the brain as the genitals during sexual stimulation. Thus, breast play is not only a physical act but also a psychological one that can affect an individual's emotional wellbeing.

For some people, their breasts hold symbolic significance in terms of femininity, motherhood, or even body image. By involving their partners in breast play, individuals may feel a deeper sense of acceptance, validation, and exploration of their bodies, leading to greater self-confidence and sexual fulfillment. Breast play can also help individuals bond with their partner through shared intimacy and trust, heightening the relationship's emotional connection.

Furthermore, breast play, like other sexual activities, can release endorphins and oxytocin, increasing feelings of pleasure and affection between partners. Oxytocin, known as the "cuddle hormone," can also promote trust and bonding, leading to a stronger emotional connection in relationships.

B. Different Ways in Which People Enjoy Breast Play

People experience pleasure in different ways, depending on individual preferences and body type. Some individuals may enjoy gentle, soft touches, while others may prefer more intense stimulation such as biting or squeezing. Additionally, some may find pleasure in nipple stimulation, whereas others may prefer stroking or licking around the areola.

It's essential to communicate and understand what type of stimulation feels pleasurable for oneself and their partner to engage in consensual breast play. Through exploration and communication, individuals can discover new sensations and ways of experiencing pleasure in their breasts.

C. The Psychological Significance of Breast Play in Sexual Relationships

Breast play can be an excellent opportunity for emotional bonding between partners, increasing feelings of intimacy and connection. As mentioned earlier, oxytocin levels increase during breast play, leading to greater feelings of trust and bonding.

In addition, engaging in pleasurable activities with one's partner can lead to increased sexual satisfaction and relationship happiness. Breast play can help promote acceptance of oneself and others, leading to deeper trust, emotional connection, and fulfillment in a relationship.

In summary, breast play is an important part of sexual exploration and can have significant psychological effects on individuals. By exploring personal preferences, communicating with one's partner, and engaging in consensual breast play, individuals can experience increased pleasure, intimacy, and emotional bonding. Breast play can help promote self-acceptance, body positivity, and sexual exploration, leading to a greater sense of emotional and psychological well-being.

It is essential to note that while breast play can be a pleasurable and meaningful experience, it is not a one-size-fits-all practice. Every individual is unique, and what feels pleasurable for one person may not be the same for another. It is vital to communicate openly with partners, establish boundaries, and respect each other's desires and preferences.

Furthermore, it's essential to understand that not all individuals may enjoy breast play. It's crucial to accept and respect personal preferences and communicate boundaries and dislikes to one's partner. Conveying discomfort or dislike towards a particular type of stimulation does not make an individual "less sexual" or "not normal." Everyone has different preferences and desires, and it's essential to respect and honor them.

Overall, breast play can be an enjoyable and meaningful part of sexual exploration. It can promote self-discovery, emotional bonding, and increased intimacy between partners. However, it's important to approach breast play with communication, respect, and an open mind to ensure a pleasurable and safe experience for all parties involved.

Chapter III.

Navigating Consent and Communication about Breast Play

Breast play can be an enjoyable and meaningful part of sexual exploration, but it's crucial to approach it with open communication and mutual respect. This chapter aims to explore the importance of communicating desires and boundaries with your partner and tips for approaching a conversation about breast play.

A. Learning How to Communicate Your Desires and Boundaries to Your Partner

Communication is key when it comes to breast play. It's essential to understand your personal preferences, desires, and boundaries before engaging in sexual activities. In this case, it's important to understand what type of stimulation feels pleasurable and what boundaries need to be established before engaging in breast play with your partner.

It's important to communicate with your partner about what you're comfortable with and what you need before moving forward with sexual activity. Establishing clear communication can lead to a sense of trust and respect between partners, which can help enhance the overall sexual experience.

When discussing desires and boundaries, it's crucial to be honest and straightforward while also being respectful and empathetic towards your partner. If you're unsure about what you want or need, take time to reflect on your desires before communicating them.

Cheryl Bach

B. Honoring Your Partner's Boundaries and Desires

Just as important as expressing your own desires and boundaries is honoring your partner's boundaries and desires. Be sure to listen actively to your partner and respect their wants and needs, even if they differ from your own.

If your partner expresses a boundary, do not pressure or attempt to coerce them into anything that makes them uncomfortable. Instead, try to understand where they're coming from and explore alternate ways of pleasuring one another that honor the limits established.

C. Best Ways to Approach a Conversation about Breast Play with Your Partner

Approaching a conversation about breast play can feel intimidating or uncomfortable for some people. However, with open communication and respect, it can be a beneficial

The Art of Breast Play

and exciting experience that enhances intimacy and sexual exploration.

One way to approach the conversation is to bring up the topic during a non-sexual moment. For example, you may want to initiate a conversation while cuddling or relaxing together, which can help create a relaxed atmosphere free from pressure.

Start the conversation by expressing your desires and curiosity about breast play. Use "I" statements to avoid sounding accusatory or judgmental towards your partner, such as "I'm interested in exploring breast play and would love to know if you're open to it."

Be sure to listen actively to your partner's response and respect any boundaries they may have. If they express interest, engage in an open dialogue about what types of stimulation feel pleasurable, and establish boundaries and safe words to ensure a mutually respectful and enjoyable experience for both parties.

It's also important to approach the conversation with an open mind and willingness to explore without judgment or shame. Breast play can be a sensitive topic for some individuals due to the societal stigma surrounding female breasts; therefore, approaching the dialogue with empathy and understanding is crucial.

If your partner expresses discomfort or resistance towards breast play, be sure to respect their boundaries and understand that not everyone enjoys this type of stimulation. Remember, sexual exploration and pleasure are unique to each individual, and it's essential to honor and respect personal preferences and desires.

In conclusion, navigating consent and communication about breast play is crucial to ensuring a pleasurable and safe experience for all parties involved. Honoring personal boundaries and desires while also approaching the conversation with respect and empathy can lead to increased intimacy, trusting relationships, and a deeper understanding of each other's sexual needs. Open communication and mutual respect are the foundations of a healthy and fulfilling sexual experience. By approaching breast play with openness and understanding, you and your partner can discover new levels of pleasure and intimacy while creating a safe and enjoyable sexual environment.

Chapter IV.

The Art of Breast Massage

Breast massage is a sensual and intimate act that can deepen sexual connection and enhance pleasure during sexual encounters. This chapter will explore the anatomy of the breasts, different techniques that can be used for breast massage, and tips for enhancing pleasure and intimacy during breast play.

A. Understanding the Anatomy of the Breasts

Before exploring the different techniques involved in breast massage, it's essential to understand the anatomy of the breasts. The breasts are composed of mammary glands and fatty tissues covered by skin. The nipple sits atop the breast, surrounded by the areola. Each breast contains a series of ducts that lead to the nipple, allowing for lactation in female-bodied individuals.

B. Different Techniques That Can Be Used for Breast Massage

There are countless techniques that can be used for breast massage. One of the best approaches is to start with light touch and gradually increase pressure or intensity as desired.

Some popular techniques include:

Circular massage: Starting from the outer edge of the breast, use your fingertips to trace a circular pattern around the breast, moving inward towards the nipple. Experiment with different levels of pressure and speed.

Squeezing: Gently squeeze the breast with your hand, releasing after a few seconds. Adjust the pressure to your partner's preference and make sure to take breaks to avoid over-stimulation.

Licking: Using your tongue, lick the nipple and surrounding areola in circular motions. Vary the pressure and speed to find what feels pleasurable for your partner.

Cupping: Place your hands around the breast, cupping gently and lifting slightly while applying pressure. Use this technique to lift and hold the breasts, or to knead and massage the flesh.

Nipple teasing: Gently tease the nipples by lightly flicking, pulling, or tracing circles around them.

It's important to communicate with your partner and ask for feedback as you perform each technique, as sensation and preference can vary greatly from person to person.

C. Tips for Enhancing Pleasure and Intimacy during Breast Massage

Breast massage can be a powerful tool for enhancing pleasure and connection during sexual encounters.

Here are some tips for maximizing the experience:

Create a comfortable and relaxing environment: Breast massage is most enjoyable when both partners feel relaxed and comfortable. Dim the lights, light some candles, and play soft music to set the mood.

Use plenty of lubrication: Using lubrication can help make the experience more comfortable and pleasurable for your partner. Experiment with different types of lubricants to find what works best for you.

Incorporate other forms of touch: Breast massage can be complemented by other forms of touch, such as kissing, caressing, and light touching of other erogenous zones.

Pay attention to your partner's reactions: Make sure to pay attention to your partner's reactions and ask for feedback. Adjust the pressure, speed, and technique as needed to ensure maximum pleasure.

Build anticipation: Breast massage can be made even more pleasurable by building anticipation beforehand. Use teasing touches and words to build excitement before moving onto breast play.

Remember to breathe: Both partners should remember to breathe deeply and regularly throughout the experience. Deep breathing can help reduce nervousness and anxiety and increase relaxation.

In conclusion, breast massage can be a powerful tool for enhancing intimacy, pleasure, and connection during sexual encounters. By taking the time to understand the anatomy of the breasts, experimenting with different techniques, and implementing tips for enhancing pleasure and intimacy, couples can create a safe, relaxing, and enjoyable experience that deepens their bond and enhances their sexual chemistry. Remember to communicate openly with your partner, listen to their feedback, and remain present in the moment to fully appreciate the pleasures of breast massage.

Chapter V.

Exploring Nipple Play

Nipples play a significant role in sexual arousal and can be a source of intense pleasure when stimulated. This chapter explores the importance of the nipples in sexual arousal, different types of nipple play techniques, and advanced techniques for more intense nipple play.

A. Understanding the Importance of the Nipples in Sexual Arousal

The nipples are highly sensitive erogenous zones that contain numerous nerve endings. When stimulated, they release oxytocin, a hormone associated with pleasure and bonding. Additionally, nipple stimulation can trigger the release of endorphins, causing a feeling of euphoria and relaxation.

For many individuals, nipple play is an essential part of foreplay and sexual encounters, leading to heightened pleasure and deeper intimacy.

B. Different Types of Nipple Play Techniques

Licking and sucking: Using your tongue and lips, lick and suck the nipples in circular motions to stimulate the nerve endings. Experiment with different levels of pressure and speed to find what feels good for your partner.

Pinching: Gently pinch the nipples between your fingers or use nipple clamps to apply pressure. Start with light pressure and gradually increase as desired.

Rolling: Using your fingers, roll the nipples between them in a back and forth motion. You can also rub the nipples in a circular motion.

Flicking: Lightly flick the nipples with your fingers or use a feather or other soft material for a more gentle touch.

Tugging: Grab the nipples and tug gently, alternating between tugging up and to the sides.

C. Advanced Techniques for More Intense Nipple Play

Nipple twister: Take the nipples between your thumb and index finger and twist them in opposite directions. This technique can be very intense, so start slow and gradually increase the pressure as desired.

Nipple pumps: Nipple pumps create suction around the nipples, increasing blood flow and sensitivity. These can be purchased at sex toy stores or online and should be used according to the manufacturer's instructions.

Temperature play: Alternating between hot and cold sensations can heighten the sensitivity of the nipples. Try using ice or a cooling gel before switching to warm oil or wax.

Sensory deprivation: Blindfolding your partner can intensify the experience and increase sensitivity to touch. This can also help create a sense of vulnerability and deeper intimacy.

It's important to communicate with your partner throughout the experience and ask for feedback to ensure that they are comfortable and enjoying themselves. Remember to take breaks if necessary to avoid over-stimulation.

In conclusion, nipple play can be a powerful tool for enhancing pleasure and connection during sexual encounters. With a variety of techniques at your disposal, you can experiment with different sensations and levels of intensity to find what works best for you and your partner. Remember to always communicate openly and listen to your partner's feedback to ensure a safe and enjoyable experience. By mastering the art of nipple play, you can take your erotic journey to new heights of pleasure, intimacy, and fulfillment.

Chapter VI.

Incorporating Toys and Accessories in Breast Play

Toys and accessories can add a new level of excitement and experimentation in breast play. They can help in exploring new sensations and can be used to complement other techniques for enhanced pleasure. This chapter provides an overview of different types of toys and accessories for breast play, safety considerations when using toys in breast play, and recommendations for buying and using toys.

A. Overview of Different Toys and Accessories for Breast Play

There are several toys and accessories that can be used in breast play.

The Art of Breast Play

Here are some of the most popular ones:

Nipple clamps: These toys apply pressure to the nipples, increasing sensitivity and arousal.

Vibrators: Vibrators can be used to stimulate the breasts and nipples, providing additional sensations and pleasurable vibrations.

White tiger balm: This is a medicated balm that creates a tingling, warming sensation on the skin. When applied to the nipples or breasts, it can create an intense sensation.

Feather ticklers: These are soft, fluffy accessories that can be used to tease and tickle the breasts and nipples, creating a playful and sensual touch.

Leather or lace corsets: These are sexy lingerie pieces that can be used to enhance the appearance of the breasts and create a seductive atmosphere.

B. Safety Considerations for Using Toys in Breast Play

When using toys and accessories in breast play, it is important to take safety into consideration.

Here are some tips to ensure a safe and enjoyable experience:

Choose high-quality toys from reputable manufacturers to ensure they are safe and effective.

Test the toy on a less sensitive area of the body before using it on the breasts to ensure that it does not cause any adverse reactions.

Be cautious with pressure and force, especially when using nipple clamps or other toys that apply pressure. Start slowly and gradually increase the intensity to avoid discomfort or injury.

Avoid using toys that may cause irritation or allergies. Always check the materials and ingredients used in the toys before using them.

Never leave the toys on for an extended period of time, as this can cause tissue damage and lead to numbness or pain.

C. Recommendations for Buying and Using Toys

When buying and using toys for breast play, it is important to choose ones that are safe and effective.

Here are some recommendations:

Choose toys made from body-safe materials such as medical-grade silicone, glass, or stainless steel.

Look for toys with adjustable pressure settings, as this will allow you to control the intensity of the stimulation.

Read reviews of products before purchasing to ensure they are effective and safe.

Use a water-based lubricant when using toys to avoid discomfort or irritation.

Communicate with your partner about their preferences and comfort levels before incorporating toys into breast play. It is important to remember that every person's body is different, and some may not be comfortable with certain types of toys or stimulation.

Experiment with the toys to find what works best for you and your partner. Try different pressures, speeds, and techniques to explore new sensations and experiences.

In conclusion, toys and accessories can be a fun and exciting way to enhance breast play. However, it is important to prioritize safety and communication throughout the experience to ensure a pleasurable and enjoyable experience. With these recommendations in mind, you can explore new horizons in your erotic journey while staying safe and comfortable.

Chapter VII.

Breast Play and Sexual Positions

Sexual positions are an essential part of any sexual encounter, as they can dictate the level of intimacy, pleasure, and connection between partners. Breast play can be incorporated into different sexual positions to enhance pleasure and fulfill the erotic potential of each position. This chapter explores how breast play can be used in different sexual positions, techniques for maximizing pleasure and connection through breast play, and ideas for experimenting with breast play during different sexual scenarios.

The Art of Breast Play

A. How Breast Play Can Be Incorporated into Different Sexual Positions

Breast play can be incorporated into a variety of sexual positions, including:

Missionary: This classic position allows for easy access to the breasts, as the receiver lies on their back with their partner on top.

Doggy-style: This position allows for a different angle of contact with the breasts, as the receiver is on all fours and their partner enters from behind.

Cowgirl: In this position, the receiver is on top, allowing them to control the pressure and angle of breast stimulation.

Spooning: This position allows for intimate contact and caressing of the breasts while lying on your side, facing your partner's back.

Standing: Breast play can also be incorporated into standing positions, such as leaning against a wall or being picked up by your partner.

B. Techniques for Maximizing Pleasure and Connection through Breast Play during Specific Sexual Positions

Each sexual position offers unique opportunities for breast play. Here are some techniques for maximizing pleasure and connection through breast play during specific sexual positions:

Missionary: During missionary, partners can experiment with different techniques such as squeezing or massaging the breasts, licking and kissing the nipples, or gently biting and nibbling the skin around the breasts. The receiver can also guide their partner's hands to focus on specific areas of the breast that feel the most pleasurable.

Doggy-style: In this position, the receiver can arch their back to push their breasts back towards their partner, allowing for more direct stimulation. The receiver can also use their hands to squeeze and massage their own breasts or guide their partner's hands to provide maximum pleasure and connection.

Cowgirl: In this position, the receiver can lean forward to allow for easier access to the breasts, or lean back to apply pressure and stimulate their own nipples with their partner's help.

Spooning: Spooning allows for intimate caressing and fondling of the breasts, with the receiver's partner able to cup and massage the breasts from behind.

Standing: During standing positions, partners can experiment with techniques such as kissing the breasts, sucking on the nipples, or gently biting and nibbling while holding the receiver up against a wall or other surface. The receiver can also wrap their legs around their partner's waist to increase intimacy and connection while engaging in breast play.

C. Ideas for Experimenting With Breast Play during Different Sexual Scenarios

Beyond exploring breast play during different sexual positions, there are many other scenarios where breast play can be incorporated into an erotic encounter, such as:

Roleplay scenarios: Different roleplay scenarios such as nurse-patient, dominant-submissive, or teacher-student, offer unique opportunities for exploring breast play in a variety of ways.

BDSM activities: BDSM activities such as nipple clamps or bondage can add a new level of intensity and pleasure to breast play.

The Art of Breast Play

Sensory play: Experimenting with different sensory experiences such as using ice cubes or feathers can elicit new sensations and stimulate the breasts in unique ways.

Mutual breast play: Partners can take turns stimulating and exploring each other's breasts, with each partner guiding the other to their preferred techniques and levels of pressure.

Oral sex: Incorporating breast play during oral sex by stimulating the breasts or nipples can add a heightened level of intensity and pleasure to the experience.

Foreplay: Using breast play as a part of extended foreplay can help build anticipation and heighten arousal for both partners.

With these ideas and techniques in mind, partners can explore the different ways in which breast play can be incorporated into their sexual encounters, creating deeper intimacy, connection, and pleasure in their erotic journey.

In conclusion, breast play can be incorporated into a variety of sexual positions and scenarios to enhance pleasure, connection, and fulfillment. By experimenting with different techniques and approaches, partners can find new ways to explore their desires, deepen their connection and intensify their mutual pleasure. Whether during missionary, doggy-style, cowgirl, spooning, standing, or in other scenarios like roleplay, BDSM activities, sensory play, oral sex or foreplay, breast play has endless possibilities for exploration and erotic discovery. So don't be afraid to experiment with different techniques, tips, and approaches to find what works best for you and your partner. With open communication, trust, and a willingness to explore and experiment, breast play can become a powerful tool for building intimacy, strengthening connections, and enhancing the pleasures of your erotic journey.

Cheryl Bach

Chapter VIII.

Breast Play and Foreplay

Breast play is an integral part of foreplay that often gets overlooked. However, taking time to explore the breasts of your partner can lead to a more fulfilling and intimate sexual experience. The sensations derived from breast play can trigger the production of oxytocin, also known as the "love hormone," which can enhance the bond between partners.

A. The Importance of Breast Play in Foreplay

Foreplay is an essential part of any sexual experience, and it is the preliminary act that helps set the mood of the scene. It's that moment where each touch is an indication of what's to come. In this regard, breast play should never be overlooked. It not only helps to ease her nerves and stimulate her senses but also to create a bond in intimacy, as the breasts are very sensitive and can produce great pleasure when touched right.

The breasts are a highly erogenous zone, and stimulation can provide immensely pleasurable experiences. Stimulation of the breasts during foreplay can create enhanced intimacy and connection between partners. Engaging in breast play ensures that the woman's mind and body are fully prepared for intercourse and that both partners are in sync regarding their desires. Overall, breast play should never be underestimated as an important part of foreplay.

B. Different Ways to Incorporate Breast Play into Foreplay

There are many different ways to incorporate breast play in foreplay, including:

The Art of Breast Play

Kissing, touching, and massaging the breasts: This physical contact can produce immense pleasure and help to set the mood for what's to come.

Teasing the nipples with the tongue: The tongue is one of the most sensitive parts of the body, and using it to tease the nipples can provide incredible pleasure.

Using oils and lotions: Adding oils or lotions to the breasts can make for a sensual and pleasurable experience. Not only does it make the breasts feel smooth and soft, but it can also increase arousal levels.

Roleplaying: Incorporating a roleplay scenario, such as pretending to be strangers and meeting for the first time, can provide an element of excitement and enhance the breast play experience.

Cheryl Bach

Using toys: Incorporating toys such as nipple clamps or vibrators can provide a new level of pleasure during breast play, and can be a great way to add a little kink to the foreplay experience.

C. Creative Techniques to Enhance the Pleasure of Breast Play during Foreplay

There are several techniques that can enhance the pleasure of breast play during foreplay, including:

Varying the intensity: Changing the intensity of the touch, from soft to hard, can create a range of sensations and keep things interesting.

Nipple twisting: Twisting and pulling on the nipples can be a very pleasurable experience for some women. However, it's important to check in with your partner and make sure she's comfortable with this level of intensity.

Sucking: Gently sucking on the nipples can create a suction sensation that can produce intense pleasure.

Massaging surrounding areas: Massaging the areas around the breasts, such as the chest and shoulders, can help to alleviate tension and enhance relaxation, which in turn enhances pleasure during breast play.

Paying attention to feedback: The most important technique when it comes to breast play is paying attention to your partner's feedback. Make sure you communicate with your partner and listen to what they enjoy so you can tailor the experience to their preferences.

In conclusion, breast play is an important aspect of foreplay that can create enhanced intimacy and connection between partners. It's essential to take the time to not only explore the physical sensations, but also to communicate with your partner and listen to their desires and feedback.

Experimenting with different techniques and incorporating different tools can keep things interesting and enhance pleasure, but it's important to always prioritize your partner's comfort and consent. By taking the time to engage in breast play and tailor the experience to your partner's preferences, you can create an unforgettable and highly fulfilling sexual experience for both partners.

Chapter IX.

The Psychology of Breast Play and Connection

A. The Role of Breast Play in Deepening Intimacy and Emotional Connection

Breasts can be an incredibly powerful source of pleasure and intimacy, oftentimes providing access to deeper psychological connections between partners. Breast play can increase dopamine and oxytocin levels, which can deepen the emotional connection between partners. This is particularly true when there is a sense of empathy and understanding between the partners.

Breast play allows you to truly connect with your partner in an intimate way and be present in the moment. Focusing on the breasts can help to take your mind off of other stresses in your life and allow for a profound bonding experience with your partner.

B. How Breast Play Can Help Foster Trust, Vulnerability, and Openness with Your Partner

Breast play can create a safe space for partners to explore their desires and connect on a deeply emotional level. The act of touching and exploring your partner's breasts can be incredibly intimate, and it requires a certain level of trust and vulnerability to open up in this way.

Additionally, breast play can help to foster a sense of openness and communication between partners. By exploring each other's bodies and discovering what feels good, partners can build a stronger connection and enhance their sexual chemistry.

When approaching breast play, it's important to communicate clearly and openly with your partner about what feels good and what doesn't. This level of communication can help to establish trust and create a safe space for both partners to fully enjoy the experience.

C. Techniques for Connecting Both Physically and Emotionally through Breast Play

There are several techniques that can help partners connect both physically and emotionally through breast play.

These techniques include:

Focusing on the sensations: Encourage your partner to focus on the sensations they are experiencing while touching and exploring your breasts. This can help to deepen the connection and bring about a greater sense of intimacy.

Making eye contact: Maintaining eye contact while engaging in breast play can help to create a deeper emotional connection and increase feelings of vulnerability and openness.

Incorporating verbal communication: Verbally communicating with your partner during breast play can help to establish trust and create a sense of emotional connection. Offer feedback on what feels good or make requests for what you'd like your partner to do.

Exploring erogenous zones: Breasts are just one of many erogenous zones on the body. Incorporating other erogenous zones, such as the neck or inner thighs, can help to deepen the physical and emotional connection during breast play.

Fostering a sense of mutual pleasure: Focus on creating a sense of mutual pleasure during breast play. Be sure to check in with your partner to make sure they are enjoying the experience and also communicate your own desires and needs.

In addition to these techniques, it's important to remember that breast play is a personal and unique experience for each individual. What feels good for one person may not feel good for another, so it's important to communicate with your partner and be receptive to their feedback.

The key to connecting both physically and emotionally through breast play is to remain present and focused in the moment. By focusing on the sensations, emotions, and desires that arise during breast play, partners can deepen their connection and enhance their overall sexual experience.

In conclusion, breast play can be a profound and meaningful experience for couples seeking to deepen their intimacy and emotional connection. By focusing on the psychological aspects of breast play, couples can create a safe space for vulnerability, trust, and openness in their sexual encounters. Techniques such as focusing on sensations, making eye contact, incorporating verbal communication, exploring other erogenous zones, and fostering mutual pleasure can all contribute to this deepened connection.

By embracing the unique experiences and desires of each partner, breast play can become a powerful tool for enhancing intimacy, fostering emotional connection, and creating a truly fulfilling erotic journey together. So take the time to explore your partner's breasts, communicate your desires and needs, and embrace the powerful emotional potential that breast play can bring to your relationship.

Chapter X.

Where to Take Your Erotic Journey

A. Understanding How Breast Play Can Fit into Your Erotic Journey

Breast play can be a powerful and transformative experience in your erotic journey, providing a new level of emotional connection and physical pleasure. Whether you are just starting out exploring your erotic journey or are seasoned in your exploration, incorporating breast play into your sexual repertoire can enhance the fulfillment and intimacy between partners.

One way breast play can fit into your erotic journey is by exploring new sensations and experiences with your partner. This could include experimenting with different techniques or incorporating toys like nipple clamps or vibrators. For those who enjoy BDSM, breast play can be a unique aspect of power exchange dynamics, helping to deepen the connection between partners.

Additionally, breast play can provide a new level of closeness and intimacy between partners inviting a deeper emotional connection and trust. This could involve exploring other aspects of your sexual desires and boundaries with open communication and consent. Some couples may choose to incorporate breast play as part of foreplay or even during non-sexual moments, such as cuddling or massages.

B. Tips for Continuing to Grow and Explore Your Sexual Desires and Boundaries

As you continue on your erotic journey, it is important to constantly reassess your desires and boundaries, while also being open and receptive to new experiences.

Here are some tips for growth and exploration in your journey:

Communicate openly: Communication is key in any sexual encounter, but especially when it comes to exploring new desires and boundaries. Be honest and open with your partner about what feels good and what doesn't, and try to remain non-judgmental and receptive to their needs as well.

Practice self-exploration: Take the time to explore your own body and desires in a safe and comfortable setting. Experiment with different techniques or toys on your own and take note of what feels good and what doesn't. This knowledge can then be communicated with your partner to enhance your sexual experiences together.

Be open to new experiences: It's important to remain open to new experiences and ideas that may arise in your erotic journey. This doesn't mean you have to say yes to everything, but be willing to listen and consider different perspectives and desires that may arise.

Embrace your sexuality: Embracing your sexuality means accepting and celebrating who you are and what you desire. This may involve letting go of shame or negative stigmas surrounding sex, and instead focusing on the positive aspects of your desires and pleasure.

C. Recommendations for Resources and Further Reading about Breast Play and Related Topics

If you're interested in diving deeper into the topic of breast play and enhancing your erotic journey, there are a variety of resources and sources of further reading available.

Here are a few possible options:

Sex-positive websites and blogs: There are many websites and blogs dedicated to sex positivity and providing information on topics such as breast play, BDSM, consent, and more. Some examples include "Bustle Sex Ed," "Kinkly," and "Sexual Alpha."

Books on sexuality: There are many books available that offer guidance on exploring your sexuality and enhancing your erotic journey. A few highly recommended titles include "The Guide to Getting It On!" by Paul Joannides, "Come As You Are" by Emily Nagoski, and "The Art of Sexual Ecstasy" by Margot Anand.

Sex therapists and counselors: If you're looking for more personalized guidance and support in exploring your sexual desires and boundaries, working with a sex therapist or counselor can be a great option. They can provide a safe and non-judgmental space to explore your personal struggles and offer clinical guidance and techniques to enhance your erotic journey.

Workshops and events: Many events and workshops focused on sexuality, kink, and BDSM can be found locally or online. These can be great opportunities to meet like-minded individuals and learn from experts on enhancing your sexual experiences.

In conclusion, breast play can be a powerful component of your erotic journey, providing a new level of emotional connection and physical pleasure. By incorporating open communication, self-exploration, and a willingness to explore new experiences, you can continue to grow and enhance your pleasure in all aspects of your sexual life. Remember to continue educating yourself about the different aspects of sexuality and exploring resources such as sex-positive websites, books on sexuality, sex therapists, and workshops or events. With patience, openness, and a willingness to explore new desires and boundaries, you can continue to deepen your connection with your partner and experience new levels of pleasure and fulfillment in your erotic journey.

Chapter XI.

Conclusion

A. Recap of the Importance of Breast Play in Sexual Relationships

Breast play is an essential aspect of sexual relationships and can provide a new level of intimacy, pleasure, and fulfillment. When executed with care and attention, breast play has the power to facilitate a deeper emotional connection between partners and can enhance overall satisfaction and pleasure in all aspects of your erotic journey.

B. How Breast Play Can Enhance Pleasure, Intimacy, and Fulfillment in Your Erotic Journey

Apart from the physical pleasure that breast play provides, it can also lead to deeper emotional connections between partners. This is because, during breast play, hormones such as oxytocin and dopamine are released, which are responsible for feelings of affection, intimacy, and bonding between partners.

Furthermore, breast play can trigger the release of endorphins, which can increase pleasure and decrease stress and anxiety. It can also stimulate the clitoris and other erogenous zones, leading to more intense and satisfying orgasms for both partners.

Breast play also provides a platform for couples to explore their boundaries and desires. When approached with open communication and consent, breast play can act as a gateway to further sexual exploration and experimentation.

Finally, incorporating breast play into your erotic journey can help enhance overall sexual and emotional fulfillment, leading to greater intimacy and a stronger bond between partners.

C. Final Thoughts on Embracing the Art of Breast Play

In conclusion, breast play is an integral component of sexual relationships and can provide a new level of intimacy, connection, and pleasure. Remember to approach breast play with open communication, consent, and a willingness to explore new desires and boundaries.

It is also helpful to continue your education and research into breast play and sexuality as a whole, as this can help to deepen your understanding and provide new insights into your erotic journey.

Remember that every individual and every couple is unique, with their own desires, boundaries, and preferences. Therefore, it is essential to approach breast play and all aspects of sexuality with an open mind and a willingness to tailor the experience to the needs and desires of yourself and your partner.

Embracing the art of breast play requires patience, communication, and a willingness to embrace vulnerability and trust. But the rewards can be immense - a stronger bond with your partner, deeper intimacy, and a more fulfilling, pleasurable erotic journey.

So don't be afraid to explore the world of breast play and embrace all that it has to offer. With care, attention, and communication, it can truly enhance your sexual experiences and bring you closer to your partner than ever before. Remember to take your time, communicate your desires and boundaries, and always prioritize the comfort and pleasure of both you and your partner.

It is my hope that this guide has helped you to gain a deeper understanding of breast play and how it can enhance your erotic journey. As you continue to explore and grow in your sexual experiences, remember to approach each new endeavor with curiosity, openness, and a desire for connection and pleasure. Wishing you all the best in your journey towards sexual fulfillment and happiness!

Cheryl Bach